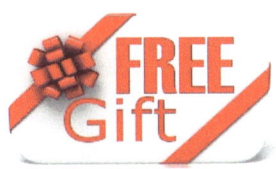

Want Priority Access to FREE eBooks Additional Materials for this Book?

As we release NEW eBooks, we offer them for FREE for a limited time. You will be the FIRST one to know when they are FREE. Join 1000's of insiders who are getting access to FREE Kindle book promotions weekly.

Click HERE for FREE additional material and FREE eBooks- www.rictamilypublishing.com

TABLE OF CONTENTS

Chapter 1: The Basics of coconut oil

Chapter 2 Coconut oil and beauty products

Chapter 3 Coconut oil for weight loss

Chapter 4 Coconut oil for pets

Chapter 5 Coconut oil snapshot

Conclusion

Review Link

Our Other Books

Dedication

Disclaimer

Copyright

Chapter 1: The Basics of coconut oil

Coconut oil is one of nature's super products that are only just starting to get the attention it deserves. Doctors all over the world have explained that Virgin Coconut oil; especially organic is one of the healthiest oil products out there. It has a fantastic amount of health benefits and there is a great deal of research to back it up. One of the best things you can do for yourself is start using coconut oil regularly in your daily routine. Before you do, though you might want to know a little bit more about the history of the fantastic and useful oil.

For more than 3800 years fruits and vegetables have been documented for use as not only eating but for use in medicine. The coconut palm has been used in a great deal of things and it seems that every year the reports about what a great help the coconut can be get better. The coconut balm has been a resource that can be sustained since those early days, it was a crop that was easy to cultivate and the harvest of the trees can be used in a variety of ways. Those who lived in tropical climates used the coconut palm for food flesh and fruit, coconut water, coconut milk and coconut oil.

The use of the oil from the coconut has been highly documented in every tropical region in the world, including South America, Central America, India, Africa and large parts of Asia. There is a document called the Ayurvedicmedicine which has been written in Sanskrit from around 1550BC where it is stated that coconut oil is great to use for the body, the mind and the spirit.

Coconut oil has even been documented as being used in WWII. In a pinch medics could use the water from young coconuts in place of a saline drip, this ability to be used saved a great many lives. After the war when rationing was still on coconut oil was used in England and the USA in place of butter.

In the 1950's however, coconut butter started to get some bad press. After centuries of being used and the benefits being seen people began to say that coconut oil was bad for you because of the saturated fat. The simple statements across the board were saturated fat is bad and that was that, anything with saturated fat was deemed bad. What those who made this campaign didn't realize is that there is a difference between the three different types of fat, they just lumped them all into one general this is bad for your health column. Everyone actually does require some fat in their diet in order to survive and be healthy.

Thanks to the modern day and technology, we have been able to start getting rid of some of the campaign stories that were spread in the 1950's. Research has shown that not all saturated fat is made the same and those which are found in coconut oil are completely unique. The way they are made up structurally because it has a chain of medium acids which are fatty. The closest comparative showing of these acids is those which can be found in Mothers milk. This unique fatty acid make up is why you will see coconut used in baby formula, Gatorade and other sports drinks and even energy bars. When you look at the ingredients on your bar or drink you can often see coconut water or oil marked down as MCT or medium chain triglycerides.

MCT's are easily digestible and that is why they are often used along with the health benefits of coconut oil. The reason that medium chain fatty acids are better is because they are processed right away and the liver converts them into energy right away. With this ease of digestion and conversion it puts less stress on the digestive system, liver and pancreas. This easier digestion also makes the rate of absorption of the minerals and nutrients faster so it is overall better for your body.

Early research in the 1950's and beyond (until recently) didn't show this easier digestion because the research was done on hydrogenated coconut oil. This process takes any fats in something and turns them into a manmade carcinogenic trans fat and trans fats are dangerous. Sadly, many of the "low" fat and "non" fat supposed healthy oils on the market today are really hydrogenated oils. These hydrogenated oils are associated with many health issues over 65 have so far been documented.

When you use coconut oil for beauty products, health products, your pets or cooking you need to use virgin coconut oil. By using virgin coconut oil you are keeping things pure and using oil that is resistant to any free radical conversion when being heated in the skillet. This resistance makes virgin coconut oil safe to cook with and use in products.

Coconut oil can be used for a great deal of things, which include (but are not limited to):

Alzheimer's

Head lice

Improves blood sugar levels

Helps with inflammation

Replacement for cooking oils

Helps with cramp pain

Removes parasites

Chapstick

Diaper salve

Weight loss

Back pain

Adrenal fatigue

Cellulite

Stress Relief

Moisturizing and cleaning leather products

Goo Gone

Nutritional supplement

Skin problems

Massage Oil

Cholesterol control

Hot flashes

Digestion

Migraines

Seasoning cookware

Relieve gallbladder pain

Acne

Asthma

Depression

Energy boost

Stretch Mark Cream

Canker sores

Moisturizer

Deodorant

Healing salve

Flaky, dry skin

Genital warts

Hair Gel/Defrizzer

Candida albicans

Lubricant

Mental Clarity

Great for dogs and cats for health

Nipple Cream

Toenail fungus

Preshave

Swimmers Ear

Eye cream

Sunscreen

Aftershave

Immune booster

Insect repellent

Chronic fatigue

Circulation/feeling cold all the time

Thrush

Seasoning animal hide drums

Herpes

Eczema

Acid

Toothpaste

Polishing Bronze

Polish Furniture

Bleeding hemorrhoids

Body scrub

Make up remover

Athlete's foot

Nosebleeds

Hair Conditioner/Deep Treatment

Chewing Gum

Autism

Mononucleosis

Bug Bites

In the next chapter we will go over some of the best beauty secrets and recipes using coconut oil.

Chapter 2 Coconut oil and beauty products

Coconut oil is great in beauty recipes. It is all natural, easy to obtain and real nourishing no matter which way you slice it. Coconut oil is especially great because it can be used on sensitive skin and for those with serious dry and flaky skin issues. In this chapter you will get some of the best and easiest recipes to use coconut oil.

The Basic whip

This basic coconut oil whip is very easy and fast to make. It has only one ingredient and that is coconut oil. It makes a rich moisturizer and that feels fantastic and even better if you want, you can add in some essential oils and have your own bath and body works thick cream.

Ingredients needed:

Coconut oil 1 cup for a single batch use more if you want a bigger batch

1 teaspoon Vitamin E (if you want)

Essential oils if you wish

How to make it:

Step 1: Place your ingredients into a large mixing bowl. Make sure that the coconut oil is in a solid state and it is great if you can use a stand mixer.

Step 2: Mix the coconut oil and anything else that you have put into the bowl on high for around 8 minutes. Use a wire whisk and keep whisking until the oil has turned into a light and airy mass.

Step 3: Spoon your fresh whip out of the bowl and into your favorite jar.

Key lime whip

Ingredients

Half cup coconut oil

1 tbsp olive oil

2 tbsp aloe vera

25 drops lime essential oil

25 drops lemon essential oil

How to make it:

Step 1: Just like with the basic whip you will place everything into the bowl. Once again make sure that the coconut oil is solid and not melted.

Step 2: Put the mixer on high and blend the ingredients and oil until it has become a light and airy texture. Start looking for this at about 3 minutes and go from there.

Step 3: Spoon the mixture into your favorite jar and secure the lid. It is best to store coconut oil, whips at room temperature, but if you live in a hot area without AC place it in the fridge.

Coconut oil hand scrub

You want to scrub your hands with a moisturizing wash this is the perfect thing for you.

Ingredients:

1/4 cup sea salt

1/4 cup organic sugar

1 tbsp coconut oil

2 tbsp raw honey

1 tbsp lemon juice

How to make it:

Step 1: First mix together the coconut oil and the honey together in a medium mixing bowl.

Step 2: In a smaller bowl you will want to blend together the salt, sugar and lemon juice. Keep blending until the whole mixture is like crumbly sand.

Step 3: Pour the blended salt mix into the honey and coconut mixture and stir together. Continue stirring the mixture until it becomes smooth.

Step 4: Store the mix in a container that is airtight preferably glass.

How to use it once it is made:

Use a small amount of the mixture, perhaps the size of a small marble and massage it into your

hand for 1 minute.

Rinse your hands off with warm water and gently pat them dry.

You can use this mixture as often as you like, but a regime or two times per week are best.

Beach Polish

Ingredients:

1/4 cup Epsom salts

2 teaspoons concentrated liquid minerals

20 drops of your favorite essential oils

1/2 cup coconut oil

1/4 cup fine ground sea salt

How to make it:

Step 1: Place the solid coconut oil into a medium sized bowl and add your salts in as well and blend very well.

Step 2: Add in your liquids and blend well until everything is perfectly blended.

Step 3: Your polish is done and you can now use it anytime you like. Store in a glass jar.

Coconut Oil Lotion Bar

Ingredients:

1 part Pure Beeswax

Essential Oils

1 part Coconut Oil

How to make it:

Step 1: In a saucepan you will want to combine the coconut oil and the beeswax together. Carefully melt it and blend as you melt. The beeswax melts more evenly if you break it into small chunks slowly.

Step 2: Once the coconut oil and beeswax are melted you will add in the essential oils.

Step 3: Pour your blend into the chosen container you have picked. You can use molds and have a free bar once done or you can chose a tin container, but that would remove the bar portion.

How to use:

If you have not used lotion bars before it can be a little difficult to use one at first. Some will bring them into the shower first and some will just use it wrong in another way. Just rub the bar onto your skin and let it slowly melt as you do, it works just like lotion.

Coconut oil eyeliner

Keeping your make up as natural as possible this is a great way to start. Eye liner is something that almost every woman uses on a day to day basis.

Ingredients:

1 - 2 capsules of activated charcoal if you want black or ½ tsp cocoa powder if you want brown

4 teaspoons aloe vera gel

2 teaspoons coconut oil

Directions

This is really easy, just mix everything up until it is smooth and store in an airtight container.

This needs to be kept dark and cool in order to keep the color and the right consistency.

Coconut Oil Lip Balm

Ingredients:

1 Tablespoon Beeswax

1 Teaspoon Red Palm Oil or Olive Oil*

1 Tablespoon Coconut Oil

*Using red palm will give your lip balm with a little bit of color

How to make it:

Step 1: Warm the coconut oil, other oil and beeswax in a double boiler system. Keep the heat low and slow as you go and melt the mixture evenly and blend.

Step 2: Continue blending for several minutes after it is melted

Step 3: Place the blended mixture into a storage container and let cool.

If you are ready to keep learning about coconut oil you will want to find what it does to help aid in weight loss.

Chapter 3 Coconut oil for weight loss

Coconut oil is great for use in cooking any kind of food you want to have but it is also fantastic for weight loss. The question you may have if you are not familiar with coconut oil is just how it manages to be so great for weight loss. In this chapter we will cover why coconut oil is fantastic for your weight loss and your overall health.

Coconut oil boosts energy levels: Since coconut oil is made up of mostly the previously mentioned medium-chain triglyceride (MCT) which can also be called lauric acid it works with your body. This fatty acid, which is needed for your body breaks down very fast compared to other fats. Since it does break down so fast and the body doesn't store MCT like it does other fats you ingest it simply uses the energy. The broken down MCT goes to your liver and the liver converts it right away to energy for your body. So, how does that help your weight loss?

journey?

More energy means that you can work out more and feel better overall. When you add a relatively small amount of coconut oil to your diet anywhere from 2 to 4 tablespoons into your diet you will get a boost of energy. It is best to consume with your morning meal and you will see a large boost in energy anywhere from 5-10% of energy for 24 hours. If you stick to this every day, you will always have that boost of energy. For most people the best way to add this coconut oil into their diet is cooking with it!

Here is one great breakfast recipe is this fantastic oatmeal:

Prep time 10 minutes

Cook time 45 minutes

Total elapsed time

55 mins

Makes:

6 servings

Ingredients

¼ cup coconut oil, measure once it is melted

1½ cups diced rhubarb

1 cup diced strawberries

1 teaspoon cinnamon

3 cups old fashioned oats

1¾ cups milk (almond milk also works)

1 teaspoon vanilla

½ cup honey

½ cup chopped walnuts

½ teaspoon salt

3 eggs

2 teaspoons baking powder

How to make it:

Step 1: Preheat your oven to 350 degrees

Step 2: Take a 9 by 13 baking dish and grease it with your favorite healthy grease, you can use coconut oil for this and then set the dish aside.

Step 3: Take a large mixing bowl and mix the dry ingredients so that will be your, baking powder, salt, oats and cinnamon and stir until they are combined.

Step 4: In a second bowl you will want to use a whisk and combine the wet ingredients so that will include yours, honey, coconut oil, milk, eggs and vanilla.

Step 5: Combine your two mixtures with a spatula. Stirring the two mixtures until they are fully combined.

Step 6: Take your rhubarb, strawberries and nuts and fold them carefully into the mixture.

Step 7: Take the blend and pour it into your baking dish that has been previously prepared.

Step 8: Bake in the oven for between 40 and 50 minutes, depending on how golden the top gets for you.

Coconut oil staves off cravings: Thanks to the MCT's that are in coconut oil that move right to the liver while they are digested you get keystones. The energy boost is helped by this and keystones naturally help to lower the cravings you will get from hunger. It is easy to know why that helps you when you are on a diet or just trying to lose a little weight. If you just keep with those 2 to 4 teaspoons of coconut oil per day in your diet, you can help to keep any large snacking impulses down between your meal times.

Burns fat: Fat burning is an important thing when you are trying to drop weight and everyone knows that. Reducing your calorie intake and raising how you burn fat is a must for weight loss and coconut oil can help with that. The raised digestion and faster nutrient absorption that coconut oil provides makes the fat cells burn better and faster with everything that you do. Coconut oil also boosts your mood and allows you to feel less stressed with its natural properties. When you feel better, have more energy and just want to do better you will do better and can do more exercise. The more exercise you do the better for your heart health and your weight loss. Coconut oil is especially good at helping to target that belly fat that can be so hard to get rid of.

Balances hormones: When you don't have the right basic set up for your body (the right fatty acids and everything else) you won't be able to get the hormones synthesize in your body properly. The MCT's in coconut oil will help the body to make hormones correctly in the way that it helps convert cholesterol and pregnenolone. So in short coconut oil will encourage your body to produce the best hormones in your body and keep you balanced.

Coconut Oil Helps The Body Absorb Nutrients faster: As mentioned before coconut oil will help your body take in nutrients faster and easier because of the improved digestion. You will absorb key vitamins such as A, D, E and K easier and better. These key vitamins are needed in your diet because they help with very important things such as cellular regeneration, healthy skin and strong bones. As well as improved mood, and brain function. Vitamin D itself is something that helps with taking in minerals like calcium, iron, zinc and magnesium. This aids in weight loss because the more efficiently that your body takes in vitamins the better it can also deal with fats and other conversions. You will have less hunger pains and more energy as well, so it is just a great motivation overall. The better you feel, the better your body will run.

Coconut Oil works to Stabilize Your Blood-Sugar: The great thing about the easy digestion of coconut oil is that when you eat it and it digests it doesn't use any enzymes for digestion. This means that your pancreas will be less stressed and it aids in the ability to produce insulin. Thanks to also being a healthy saturated fat, coconut oil also allows cells to bind easier with insulin during the digestion process. Due to this your body better receives the glucose it needs as it needs it.

It can be overwhelming when you first start adding coconut oil into your diet for the purposes of weight loss. There is a lot of information to take in and sometimes you can lose track of how much you should be taking. The one thing to remember about coconut oil is not to go overboard, if you do the fat levels may start to counteract your weight loss goals.

If you don't want to cook with the coconut oil you can take it 20 minutes before meal times and spread it out over each meal. You can melt the coconut oil into hot water or tea. Or if you prefer, you can simply put it in your mouth and allow it to melt. The amounts that you should have for weight loss are:

- 90-130 lbs, use 1 TBL coconut oil per meal
- 131-180 lbs, use 1.5 TBL coconut per meal
- Over 180 lbs, use 2 TBL coconut oil per meal

The next chapter will cover what coconut oil does for our pets!

Chapter 4 Coconut oil for pets

Coconut oil is not only great for people, but it can be used for animals as well. Most of the same benefits for people translate right to our furry friends as well which include:

•	The coconut is great for nutrition and the whole fruit can be used. This includes the juice, flesh and oil. The coconut oil of course, as we have covered is the best for you with the most benefit and is the easiest to feed to animals. The 90% saturated fat content of coconut oil also has antimicrobial, antibacterial, and antifungal uses and properties.

•	Coconut oil will help bump up antioxidants and boost the absorption of other minerals.

•	Coconut oil has MCFA's which will give a great deal of health benefits for your pet friends.

When you use coconut oil with a healthy diet for your pets, you will see that their digestion is improved and their coats look fantastic. If they do have the instance of getting an infection you will see it cure faster and skin conditions will be less prevalent. When animals like dogs and cats who have a high meat diet live in the wild, they naturally take in more saturated fat than we do, but the kibble diets, they have with us, take most of that out, coconut oil can add it back in on a healthy level.

The great thing about using coconut oil for dogs and cats is that it can be used both externally and internally. It will clear up skin rashes and infections. It can be used topically to clean cuts as well it can also be used to help deodorize your dog's skin and help them smell better without giving them a full bath.

Many herbal remedies that you try to give to your pets are hard to get them to eat. Coconut oil however is something that most dogs and cats too will love to eat. You can probably just offer it on a spoon and watch them eat it or melt it and pour it over their food. The light nut taste makes it tasty for them just like it does with people. The research being done on coconut oil use for pets is getting more vets to actually recommend a regime or the daily coconut oil use to keep dogs and cats healthy.

The key to use coconut oil for pets knows how much you should give them. Luckily that dose is pretty easy to figure out. Give one teaspoon of coconut oil per every 10 pound of dog or you can transfer that to one tablespoon per 30 pounds of dog. When you first start giving coconut oil work with about 1/3 of the recommended dose and slowly increase that over a month's time. If you just start with the full dose right away you can cause your dog to have some symptoms of illness.

Cats on the other hand should get one teaspoon of coconut oil a day as long as they are over 6 months of age. Again, like with the dog you will start with about 1/3 of the recommended dose and then slowly add in more over a month of time.

If you want to help keep fleas away from your dog, especially during the flea season you can brush their coats with coconut oil every two weeks during the high flea times. This is a great natural remedy to keeping fleas away from your beloved pet without using high

chemical topicals.

When skin conditions, crop up you can rub coconut oil into the problem as it appears. Continue to use a daily regime until you see the issue clearing up.

Puppies who are just starting to wean can use the extra saturated fat and you can add a little coconut oil over their first solid meals to help keep them safe, healthy and getting enough nutrients.

The final thing to know when feeding your beloved pet's coconut oil is which kind to get them. The best coconut oil to use is an Organic Virgin coconut oil and one of the bets suppliers of these coconut oils is Tropical Traditions. You can get several levels from them, gold, green label or expeller pressed. The key is to just use unrefined coconut oil for your pets.

In the final chapter we will cover a snap shot of what coconut oil is great for.

Chapter 5 Coconut oil snapshot

In this final chapter, we will take a fast look at what coconut oil can do for you. This is a snapshot of health benefits and why coconut oil works to help you. It is a simple fact that coconut oil is a super food and a super herbal remedy.

Oral Health: If you prefer natural health this is a great solution to help keep your mouth

healthy. There are a lot of commercial toxic choices you can use, but they have chemicals. Coconut oil can be used as toothpaste and has been proven to harden enamel and keep your mouth from developing sores.

Fungal Treatment: Since coconut oil is super it can be used for a lot of external fungal issues but also internal. You can use coconut oil for athlete's foot and ring worm but you can also use it to help with yeast infections and Candida. Every Candida diet out there has a dose of coconut oil listed as something you need to take.

Digestive Aid: As we have covered throughout this book coconut oil is easy to digest and it aids in the digestion of other food items as well. The saturated fats will help with constipation, acid reflux and indigestion. There has been research done which also shows that it can help with serious issues such as crohn's disease and ulcertative colitis.

Nutrient Absorption: Coconut oil will help your body take in the nutrients it needs easier as we have covered throughout the book. The reason this is good is because the proper nutrients will help your body in the long run and reduce the chance of developing long term chronic diseases such as: Some forms of cancer, pancreatic issues, gallbladder problems, obesity and crohn's disease.

Energy Booster: Never forget that coconut oil will boost your energy and will do that over an entire day. It not only will boost your physical energy, but your mental energy as well. This is great when you need to focus or work out!

Weight Loss: As we covered in chapter 3 coconut oil is perfect for weight loss programs. When you combine the nutrient absorption, anti-fungal properties and energy boosting properties you get everything that you need for success. The older we get, the harder it is to lose weight because the metabolism naturally begins to slow and the organs in our bodies can feel the stress of added weight. When you take coconut oil boosts your metabolism naturally and kicks that weight loss into gear as long as you focus on a balanced diet, exercise plan and coconut oil added in.

Allergy Relief: Allergies are something that over 50 million Americans suffer from and more find out every day. Taking medicine that helps, but is another chemical in your body is something that many don't want to do so they suffer. Coconut oil can help with allergies in a natural way! Coconut oil is best in aiding in fighting food allergies such as, soy, gluten, wheat, dairy and peanuts. Using coconut oil can counteract reactions to these. However, if you have food allergies you should be aware that in some rare cases people can be allergic to coconut oil so if you don't know proceed with caution in your first use.

Cold and Flu relief: Since coconut oil has what is called the trifecta of anti-viral, anti-fungal, and anti-microbial components which also includes capric acid, lauric acid and caprylic acid it will boost your immunity. Don't use butter and instead use coconut oil in your cooking and

keep the flu from taking hold in your body. If you have the flu already just start adding doses of coconut oil into your tea and you can shorten the life span of the virus. You will also notice that coconut oil will help with your sore throat, fever chills and any inflammation that you have in your body.

Pain Relief: Coconut oil is a fantastic way to help aid in pain relief naturally. Due to all those great properties that we mentioned above. Not only will it help with cold and flu pains, but it will naturally fight, joint pain, headaches migraines and the pain from arthritis. Many Doctors who treat rheumatoid arthritis and other long term chronic pain conditions have started to look at the uses of coconut oil in fighting the pain and inflammation which is associated with the conditions. The properties within the coconut oil fight the pain and also naturally lubricate the muscles and joints of the body. When used as a topical rub it will naturally increase the blood supply to the area you are using it on. When you promote healthy circulation you also create better flexibility for your body which will aid the body and reduce pain all over.

Protect your skin: Helping against skin problems is perhaps the one best known area that coconut oil has become famous for. Whether you are using it in beauty products or just along straight from the jar coconut oil helps. It is an effective sunscreen, great for moisture, shaving cream, deodorant, diaper rash, scar reduction, stretch mark cream, and age spot removal and make up removal. The more you get used to using coconut oil the more you will find you don't need commercial products that are heavy in chemicals in your life. The more chemicals you can take out of your regime the healthier you will be overall.

The bottom line about coconut oil is that you can use it for almost anything. It truly is a miracle and it is GMO free and sustainable so it is healthy for the planet. Use this book as a quick reference anytime you find yourself reaching for something that is chemical to see if you could instead use coconut oil. In closing here is one more fantastic coconut oil recipe to add to your arsenal.

Carrot Cake Granola

Gluten free and Vegan

Prep time: 10 mins

Cook time: 25 mins

Total elapsed time: 35 mins

Ingredients:

1 full cup favorite nuts

1/4 cup of maple syrup

1/2 cup of coconut you can use shreds or shavings if you want

1 cup grated or carrots (shredded)

1 cup additional chosen nuts such as pecans

1 teaspoon cinnamon, ground is best

2 cups natural oats (use gluten free oats if you want it gluten free)

1/2 teaspoon of salt, sea salt is the best

1/4 cup coconut oil, melted down

1/8 teaspoon nutmeg the ground is best

1/2 cup fresh raisins

1/4 teaspoon ginger, ground is best

How to make it:

Step 1: Pre-heat oven to 350 degrees F.

Step 2: Combine in a medium bowl, all of the ingredients first combining the dry and then adding in the wet. Blend with a spatula until well blended.

Step 3: Use a baking sheet and spread the mixture onto it and bake in the oven for 25 minutes. Half way through the bake, remove the sheet and stir or flip the mixture.

Conclusion

Thank you again for downloading this book!

I hope this book was able to help you to understand all of the fantastic benefits of coconut oil.

The next thing you need to do is put this information to use and enjoy that wonder oil!

Review Link

If you enjoyed this book, we would really appreciate it if you could leave us a positive REVIEW?

P.S. **You can CLICK HERE to go directly to the book page** and leave your review and/or purchase our other books above. Alternatively, you can copy and paste this address into your browser --- http://amzn.to/1wCj3OE

Our Other Books

Amish Mail-Order Bride Romance Series: The Ad

Anti-Cancer Diet: The Ultimate Guide in Fighting Cancer, Lowering Cancer Risk and Achieving Optimum Health

Best Pets For Children: Ten Tips on Care and Proper Choice for Your Child

Bodyweight Exercises: Training to Build Muscle and Lose Fat - Beginner to Advanced Routines to Strengthen Your Core

Chakras for Beginners: The Ultimate Guide to Balancing Chakras, Radiating Positive Energies and Strengthening Auras

Ebola: 10 Things You Need to Know About: Facts about the Virus, Symptoms, Quarantine and Prevention

Financial Freedom: Ultimate Guide to Achieve Wealth, Attain Success and Manage Your Debt

Funeral Planning: 25 Essentials: The Ultimate Guide for Selecting Funeral Homes, Obituaries and Funeral Directors

Gilgamesh - King in Quest for Immortality: An Extra-Biblical Proof for the Genesis Flood

Gilgamesh and Sumerian 2-in-1 Christian Box Set: Biblical History: The True Nature of Intelligence; Gilgamesh: King in Quest of Immortality

Gout Cure: Your Ultimate and Comprehensive Guide in Treating Gout

Herbal Soap Making: How to Make Homemade Soaps that clean and Nurture the Body

Habit Stacking + Productivity Power: Your Daily Guide to Habit Stacking, Preventing Procrastination and Developing Successful Skills

Hillary 2016: A Lifetime in the Making

Holy Land Collection: Israel vs. The World: The Apple of God's Eye in the End of Time; and Jesus, Jews & Jerusalem: Past, Present and Future of the City

ISRAEL vs. THE WORLD: The Apple of God's Eye in the End Times

Jesus, Jews & Jerusalem: Past, Present and Future of the City of God

Liver Cleanse and Detox Diet: The Ultimate Guide to Cleansing the Body, Eliminating Toxins and Losing Weight!

Mediterranean Diet for Beginners: Cuisine Cookbook Recipes for Shredding Fat and Weight Loss

Minecraft: The Video Game about Breaking and Placing Blocks

Negative Emotions: Your Personal Guide in Controlling Anger, Managing Stress and Overcoming Fear

Overcoming Porn Addiction: A 10 Step Journey to Overcoming Internet Sexual Addiction through Jesus

Paleo and Grain-Free Diet for Beginners: Cookbook Recipes Using a Slow Cooker for Weight Loss

Pilates and Bodyweight Exercises: 2-in-1 Fitness Box Set: Shred Fat, Look Great

Pilates for Beginners: The Essential Guide to Total Body Fitness, Strong Muscles and Lean Body

Slimming Secrets and Weight Lose: Health, Fitness, and Diet Secrets for the New You

Stop Negative Self-Talk Today: Quotes and Secrets to Positive Thinking That Will Heal Your Soul

Stop Self-Sabotaging and Shift Your Paradigm to Success: Your Ultimate Guide to Living the Life You Always Wanted

Sumerian Culture: The Nature of True Intelligence: Musings on the Ancient Sumerian Culture From a Christian Perspective

Teeth Healing through Oil Pulling: The Complete Guide in Natural Oral Care through the Benefits of Oil Pulling

Wearable Technology: Discover 20 Trends and Interactive Mobile Sensor Devices to Include Medical, Wearable and Children's Devices

Wedding Planning - 25 Essentials: The Ultimate Guide for Selecting Dresses, Cakes and Decorations on a Budget

Dedication

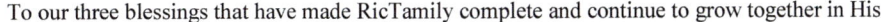

To our three blessings that have made RicTamily complete and continue to grow together in His

Loving embrace.

Disclaimer

The information in this book is in no way intended as medical advice. This book is not meant to be used, nor should it be used, to diagnose or treat any medical condition. The author disclaims responsibility for any adverse health effects that come in combination with the use of methods and suggestions presented in the book. The publisher and author are not responsible for any health or allergy needs that may require medical supervision and are not liable for any damages or negative consequences from any treatment, action, application or preparation, to any person reading or following the information in this book.

THE END